THE DIABETES CODE JOURNAL

DR. JASON FUNG

WITH RECIPES BY ALISON MACLEAN

THE
DIABETES
CODE
JOURNAL

The Official Workbook
for Reversing Type 2 Diabetes
Through Healthy Eating
and Fasting

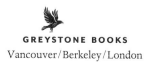

GREYSTONE BOOKS
Vancouver/Berkeley/London

"Knowing is not enough; we must apply. Willing is not enough; we must do."

BRUCE LEE

The Diabetes Code Journal is not about magical thinking.

It's about doing the hard, day-to-day work of changing your diet and lifestyle to help reverse the process of hyperinsulinemia, with the goal of putting type 2 diabetes into remission.

Remission? Is that even possible?

YES.

Greystone Books Ltd.
greystonebooks.com

Cataloguing data available from Library and Archives Canada
ISBN 978-1-77840-096-4 (pbk.)
ISBN 978-1-77840-097-1 (epub)

Editing by James Penco
Proofreading by Alison Strobel
Cover and text design by Fiona Siu

Printed and bound in China on FSC® certified paper at Shenzhen
Reliance Printing. The FSC® label means that materials used for the
product have been responsibly sourced.

Greystone Books thanks the Canada Council for the Arts, the British
Columbia Arts Council, the Province of British Columbia through the
Book Publishing Tax Credit, and the Government of Canada for
supporting our publishing activities.

Canada

  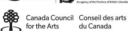

Greystone Books gratefully acknowledges the xʷməθkʷəy̓əm (Musqueam),
Sḵwx̱wú7mesh (Squamish), and səlilwətaɬ (Tsleil-Waututh) peoples on
whose land our Vancouver head office is located.

Medical disclaimer: This book is for general informational and educational purposes
only. It is not intended to constitute or substitute for medical advice, counseling,
the practice of medicine, the provision of health care, diagnosis, treatment, or the
creation of a clinical relationship between a patient and physician and/or facility.
Readers should consult their medical or health professional before adopting any of
the suggestions in this book or drawing personal medical conclusions from it. The
author and publisher specifically disclaim all responsibility for any liability, loss, or
risk, personal or otherwise, which is incurred as a consequence, directly or indirectly,
of the use and application of any of the contents of this book.

CONTENTS

THE SUGAR BOWL

Type 2 diabetes (and its precursor, prediabetes) is essentially a disease where your body has too much sugar in it. Think of a sugar bowl. If you consistently put in more than you take out, it gradually fills up. Eventually, the bowl will be so full that when you put in more sugar, it will spill over.

The same situation exists in the human body. You need energy to power your body—your heart, lungs, brain, and kidneys (via your basal metabolic rate) and your muscles (via exercise). When you eat, you put energy into your body, which can be either used or stored. You store energy in the form of glucose (a type of sugar) or body fat. When you are not eating, your body uses energy from its stored sources (glucose or body fat).

What happens in type 2 diabetes? If you are steadily putting more glucose into the body than you are taking out, your body eventually fills up, just like that sugar bowl. The next time you eat, that glucose will spill over into the blood. The blood glucose level rises, which is the defining feature of type 2 diabetes.

The problem is not simply that the blood has too much glucose, but that the entire body does too. Some medications, like insulin, simply move the excess glucose from the blood into the body. This lowers the blood glucose but not the overall glucose in the body. The excess glucose is changed into fat; the medication causes weight gain. If you were to stop taking the medication, the glucose would come back out from its storage site—making it a temporary improvement at best.

To solve the problem of excess sugar, you must get rid of it, not simply hide it away where it can't be seen. Otherwise, it's like hiding spoiled food under the sink instead of throwing it out. You can pretend your kitchen is clean, but eventually it begins to smell really, really bad. You need to throw it out, not hide it.

Framing the problem of type 2 diabetes as an excess of glucose in the body is useful because the solution becomes immediately obvious. Get rid of the excess sugar. Don't hide it away. Too much glucose in the blood is toxic, as is too much glucose in the body. If untreated, all that excess sugar in your body rots your organs. Type 2 diabetes increases the risk of heart disease, stroke, cancer, infection, blindness, kidney disease, fatty liver disease, and so much more.

"Minds, like diapers,
need occasional changing."

KAREN CUSHMAN,
THE BALLAD OF LUCY WHIPPLE

"The best of all medicines
is resting and fasting."

BENJAMIN FRANKLIN

HOW TO REVERSE TYPE 2 DIABETES NATURALLY

Many people believe that type 2 diabetes is irreversible. This is not true, according to the American Diabetes Association (ADA). In 2021, the ADA defined the clinical criteria for remission of type 2 diabetes—confirming that under certain conditions, it is indeed a reversible disease.

But taking medications generally does not lead to remission. Since type 2 diabetes is largely a dietary and lifestyle disease, remission is only possible by fixing those dietary and lifestyle issues. Drugs can't cure a dietary disease.

Think of your car. Suppose you fueled up at a gas station three times a day. If your gas tank was full but you still kept pumping gas into it, it would overflow. What would you do? I'll tell you what you *wouldn't* do: keep pumping gas! The solution? Stop putting in more gas—or drive around to burn the gas off.

The same situation happens with type 2 diabetes. If your glucose stores are full, but you keep putting more sugar into them, the glucose will overflow into your blood. The solution?

1. Put less sugar in

2. Burn the sugar off

That's it! The best part? It's all natural and completely free. No drugs. No surgery. No cost.

STEP 1: PUT LESS SUGAR IN

All foods are composed of three main macronutrients:

1. Carbohydrates—sugars, mostly glucose
2. Proteins—composed of amino acids
3. Fats—triglycerides

Low-Carbohydrate Diets

Some foods raise the blood glucose more than others, based partially on their macronutrient composition. Carbohydrates are chains of sugars, mostly glucose. Therefore, when you eat carbohydrates (glucose), your blood glucose tends to rise. How much it rises is reflected in the "glycemic index"—a scale that measures how much specific foods affect the average person's blood glucose, and which only applies to carbohydrate-containing foods.

Proteins are made of chains of amino acids, and fats are composed of fatty acids called triglycerides. When you eat foods composed mostly of proteins and fats, your blood glucose does not tend to rise, because you are not eating glucose. If you suffer from high levels of blood glucose, then it is logical to eat foods that tend not to raise your blood glucose. That is, in this situation, a diet low in carbohydrates is preferable.

A 2019 consensus report by the American Diabetes Association agrees,[1] stating that "reducing overall carbohydrate intake for individuals with diabetes has demonstrated the most evidence for improving glycemia." The American Heart Association[2] echoes this

1   Alison B. Evert et al., "Nutrition Therapy for Adults With Diabetes or Prediabetes: A Consensus Report," *Diabetes Care* 42, no. 5 (2019): 731–754. https://doi.org/10.2337/dci19-0014

2   Joshua J. Joseph et al., "Comprehensive Management of Cardiovascular Risk Factors for Adults With Type 2 Diabetes: A Scientific Statement From the American Heart Association," *Circulation* 145, no. 9 (2022): e722–e759. https://doi.org/10.1161/CIR.0000000000001040

advice, stating that "very low-carbohydrate...diets yield a greater decrease in A1C [a type of blood sugar test], more weight loss and use of fewer diabetes medications in individuals with diabetes."

STEP 2: BURN THE SUGAR OFF

How can you burn off excess glucose?

1. Exercise
2. Fasting

Exercise

Exercise increases the energy—especially the blood glucose—used by your muscles. Move more. This is not particularly novel or controversial.

Fasting

Fasting is the literally the oldest dietary therapy known, and it has been practiced throughout human history. "Fasting" is any time that you are not eating. This is the simplest and surest method to force your body to burn excess sugar. Your body—your brain, heart, lungs, kidneys, and other organs—needs energy, and when you are not eating, it will find this energy by burning stored fuel: glucose.

When you eat, your body *stores* food energy. When you fast, your body *burns* food energy. Lengthening your fasting periods allows you to burn off the stored sugar.

For more on the science of type 2 diabetes remission, read my book *The Diabetes Code*, to which this journal is a companion.

"The most difficult thing is the decision to act.
The rest is merely tenacity."

AMELIA EARHART

PRINCIPLES OF THE LOW-CARBOHYDRATE DIET

If your body has too much glucose, then you should eat less glucose (carbohydrates). Eat more proteins and fats instead.

GENERAL PRINCIPLES

1. Sugar: Eliminate as much as possible

2. Refined and starchy carbs: Eliminate as much as possible, since these are easily digested to glucose and therefore raise blood glucose quickly

3. Green vegetables (grown above ground): Eat as much as you like

4. Fruit: Eat in moderation. Berries are the best; other sweet fruits contain much higher levels of fructose which, like high-fructose corn syrup, can be bad for type 2 diabetes

5. Natural protein-containing foods: Avoid processed meats like sausages, hot dogs, and bologna. Eat natural meats, fish, and shellfish to satiety

6. Natural fats: Eat more natural fats found in meat, dairy, olive oil, and avocados

7. Sweeteners: Avoid, as the sweetness may stimulate appetite and cravings

8. Alcohol: Reduce; try to drink dry wines (which have the lowest sugar content)

EMPHASIZE THESE FOODS

1. Non-starchy vegetables
2. Proteins
3. Natural fats

AVOID THESE FOODS

1. Starchy foods
2. Sugary foods
3. Refined carbohydrates

"A little starvation can really do more for the average sick man than can the best medicines and the best doctors."

MARK TWAIN

PRINCIPLES OF
INTERMITTENT FASTING

When you eat, you store calories. You can't store calories and burn calories at the same time. Only not eating (fasting) allows stored calories to be burned, so give your body the time it needs to burn off those calories. As your stores of glucose and body fat go down, you can reverse your type 2 diabetes.

How long to fast? Your fast can be almost any length, but the two most popular regimens are a 16-hour fasting period and a 24-hour fasting period.

A 16-hour fasting period corresponds to an 8-hour eating window and is often called Time-Restricted Eating (TRE), or the 16/8 fasting protocol.

16-Hour Fast, 6 Days/Week

	Monday	Tuesday	Wednesday	Thursday	Friday	Saturday	Sunday
Breakfast 7 AM							✓
Lunch 12 PM	✓	✓	✓	✓	✓	✓	✓
Dinner 7:30 PM	✓	✓	✓	✓	✓	✓	✓

In a 24-hour fasting regimen, you eat one single meal in a day, which is often called One Meal a Day (OMAD). You may choose any time to eat, and many people choose an early dinner / late lunch as their meal.

24-Hour Fast, 3 Days/Week

	Monday	Tuesday	Wednesday	Thursday	Friday	Saturday	Sunday
Breakfast 7 AM	✓		✓		✓		✓
Lunch 12 PM	✓		✓		✓		✓
Dinner 7:30 PM	✓	✓	✓	✓	✓	✓	✓

"Nothing in the world can take
the place of persistence. Talent will not...
Genius will not... Education will not... Persistence
and determination are omnipotent."

CALVIN COOLIDGE

HOW TO MEASURE YOUR
BLOOD GLUCOSE

How do you know if your blood glucose is too high? You won't, unless you measure it—making measurement a critical part of getting better. This principle is called biofeedback, and it is the key to improving your performance.

Suppose you were to practice shooting free throws in basketball. Each time you threw, you would see the result—and get feedback on whether you had thrown the ball too hard, too soft, too high, too low, or off-target. Over time, you would adjust and gradually improve. That's possible because you get immediate feedback: Did the shot go in or not?

Apply this to type 2 diabetes. When you eat certain foods, you don't know how your blood glucose is reacting unless you measure it. A blood test called the hemoglobin A1C measures only the three-month average of your glucose—but do you remember what foods you ate three months ago? What if you practiced basketball for months with no idea of how you were doing, except that every three months a coach walked in and said, "You are doing poorly, on average." Not very useful, is it?

Today's technology allows for personalized medicine. You can measure your blood sugar directly in response to the foods you've just eaten. Keep a food journal and check how your eating affects your blood sugar. Over time, you will understand to which foods your body reacts well, and to which foods it does not.

There are two main ways to check your blood glucose. A glucometer measures a drop of blood obtained by pricking your finger. Each time you measure your blood glucose, you'll need to poke your finger, which is a disadvantage.

A continuous glucose monitor (CGM) uses a sensor with a very thin needle inserted into your arm, which can stay in place for two weeks at a time. You can check your blood glucose by scanning the sensor with your smartphone as often as you'd like, without further pokes.

"We first make our habits,
then our habits make us."

ATTRIBUTED TO JOHN DRYDEN

WHY JOURNAL?

Journaling is one of the simplest things you can do to keep your-self accountable, stay on track toward your goals, and guide your-self to success.

Keep this journal by your bedside table. Each night, before you brush your teeth, take just five minutes to reflect upon your day. We are trying to *build healthy habits* by consciously evaluating and reflecting. Over time, this becomes a habit, and that's when the magic starts. Habits don't take extra effort. Habits don't require thinking. Habits aren't difficult. The benefits accrue over years, or even decades.

You don't have to think about brushing your teeth because it's a habit; it doesn't require willpower. But building a habit is hard work—and this journal can help.

The key to behavior change is consistency. A little bit done consistently day after day soon adds up. Years ago, during medical school, I started skipping breakfast because I was tired and wanted to sleep. I saved an extra thirty minutes because I no longer needed to make breakfast, eat it, and clean up the dishes. I did this every day, and it soon became a habit.

Every week, I saved 3.5 hours of time. Every month, I saved 15 hours. Every year, I saved 182 hours. Over the last twenty years, I saved about 3,640 hours. All because of a habit that I cultivated years ago and haven't thought about much. That time I could spend however I wished—sleeping, relaxing, or writing books.

The secret to your future lies hidden in your daily routine.

"All progress takes place outside the comfort zone."

MICHAEL JOHN BOBAK

HOW TO USE THIS JOURNAL

Each week will start with a weekly challenge to push you out of your comfort zone. Dare yourself to do better. Think about the challenge and set your goal for the week. Then write it down.

Each day thereafter, the journal will present you with a quote or a thought. Reflect briefly upon how it applies to your life.

Empty the Sugar Bowl
(Put Less Sugar In / Burn the Sugar Off)
Record everything you ate that day, and how long you fasted. Jot down how you increased your amount of movement. Write down how your blood glucose responded. Was it what you expected? Was it higher or lower? What foods spiked your blood glucose? What foods didn't?

Reflect
Now reflect on your day. Focus on the positives, the things you did well. Recognize the things that you could have been done better, but don't beat yourself up over them. They are simply things that you can improve upon. There's always tomorrow!

Gratitude
End your day by reflecting upon a single moment that felt great. Realize that every day is precious because of these special moments.

Order: Change the order that you eat your meals by eating the carbs last. That way, you can fill up on healthy proteins and fats first.

My weekly goal–Order:
Every day this week, I will eat the carbs last.

Today I ate:
Tuna fish on salad
Hamburger with side of mashed potatoes

Today I fasted from 7 PM **until** 11 AM

Total fasting period: 16 hours

Today I moved by:
Running—30 minutes
Yoga—20 minutes

Today my blood glucose was: in the 100 range—making progress!

REFLECTIONS

What I did well:
Fasted for a good 16 hours today—felt less hunger
Ate the carbs last

What I could improve:
Could have switched my potatoes for a less-starchy vegetable

Why today was great:
Enjoyed a hot bath

The greater danger for most of us lies not in setting our aim too high and falling short, but in setting our aim too low and achieving our mark.

MICHELANGELO

How this quote applies to me: I will aim to get off all insulin in three months by reducing my carb intake. I may not reach it, but I will try my best.

Today I ate:

Oatmeal, eggs, coffee with sugar

Chicken sandwich, french fries

Lamb stew, potatoes, carrots

Today I fasted from 7 PM **until** 10 AM

Total fasting period: 15 hours

Today I moved by:

Running—30 minutes

Yoga—30 minutes

Today my blood glucose was: OK, but not great.

REFLECTIONS

What I did well:

I stuck to my fasting schedule

My food choices were OK

What I could improve:

I took one teaspoon of sugar in my coffee—tomorrow I will use only half a teaspoon

I'll swap the fries for a salad next time

Why today was great:

I saw my friend John at work today. Haven't talked to him in ages!

MY
JOURNAL

These are foods that spike my blood glucose, which I should AVOID:

....
....
....
....
....
....
....
....
....
....
....
....
....
....
....
....
....
....
....
....
....
....
....
....
....

These are foods that don't spike my blood glucose, which I should PRIORITIZE:

WEEK 1

Journaling: Fill in your journal
every day this week.

My weekly goal—Journaling: ....

....

Today I ate: ....

....

....

....

Today I fasted from .... **until** ....

Total fasting period: ....

Today I moved by: ....

....

....

Today my blood glucose was: ....

REFLECTIONS

What I did well:

....

....

What I could improve:

....

....

Why today was great:

....

....

I'm taking small steps,
'Cause I don't know where I'm going.
LOUIS SACHAR

How this quote applies to me: ....

....

Today I ate: ....

....

....

....

Today I fasted from .... **until** ....

Total fasting period: ....

Today I moved by: ....

....

....

Today my blood glucose was: ....

REFLECTIONS

What I did well:

....

....

What I could improve:

....

....

Why today was great:

....

....

A journey of a thousand miles
must begin with a single step.
LAO TZU

DAY 3

How this quote applies to me: ....

....

Today I ate: ....

....

....

....

Today I fasted from .... **until** ....

Total fasting period: ....

Today I moved by: ....

....

....

Today my blood glucose was: ....

REFLECTIONS

What I did well:

....

....

What I could improve:

....

....

Why today was great:

....

....

Today I will do what others won't, so tomorrow I can accomplish what others can't.
JERRY RICE

How this quote applies to me: ....
....

Today I ate: ....
....
....
....

Today I fasted from .... **until** ....

Total fasting period: ....

Today I moved by: ....
....
....

Today my blood glucose was: ....

REFLECTIONS

What I did well:
....
....

What I could improve:
....
....

Why today was great:
....
....

For those who are willing to
make an effort, great miracles and
wonderful treasures are in store.
ISAAC BASHEVIS SINGER

How this quote applies to me: ....

....

Today I ate: ....

....

....

....

Today I fasted from .... **until** ....

Total fasting period: ....

Today I moved by: ....

....

....

Today my blood glucose was: ....

What I did well:

....

....

What I could improve:

....

....

Why today was great:

....

....

Let food be thy medicine
and medicine be thy food.
HIPPOCRATES

How this quote applies to me: ....

....

Today I ate: ....

....

....

....

Today I fasted from .... **until** ....

Total fasting period: ....

Today I moved by: ....

....

....

Today my blood glucose was: ....

REFLECTIONS

What I did well:

....

....

What I could improve:

....

....

Why today was great:

....

....

The greatest mistake you can make in life is to be continually fearing you will make one.

ELBERT HUBBARD

DAY 7

How this quote applies to me: ....
....

Today I ate: ....
....
....
....

Today I fasted from .... **until** ....
Total fasting period: ....
Today I moved by: ....
....
....

Today my blood glucose was: ....

What I did well:
....
....

What I could improve:
....
....

Why today was great:
....
....

Great job! You finished one full week of journaling.

You are well on your way to building healthy habits
that can last a lifetime.

Keep going.

You've got this.

WEEK 2

Clean eating: Stick to your eating
principles closely this week.
Eat natural, unprocessed foods.

DAY 1

My weekly goal—Clean eating: ....

....

Today I ate: ....

....

....

....

Today I fasted from .... **until** ....

Total fasting period: ....

Today I moved by: ....

....

....

Today my blood glucose was: ....

REFLECTIONS

What I did well:

....

....

What I could improve:

....

....

Why today was great:

....

....

Just keep swimming.
DORY, *FINDING NEMO*

How this quote applies to me: ....
....

Today I ate: ....
....
....
....

Today I fasted from .... **until** ....
Total fasting period: ....
Today I moved by: ....
....
....

Today my blood glucose was: ....

REFLECTIONS

What I did well:
....
....

What I could improve:
....
....

Why today was great:
....
....

I never dreamed about
success. I worked for it.
ESTÉE LAUDER

DAY 3

How this quote applies to me: ....

....

Today I ate: ....

....

....

....

Today I fasted from .... **until** ....

Total fasting period: ....

Today I moved by: ....

....

....

Today my blood glucose was: ....

What I did well:

....

....

What I could improve:

....

....

Why today was great:

....

....

There are only two options:
make progress or make excuses.
TONY ROBBINS

How this quote applies to me: ....
....

Today I ate: ....
....
....
....

Today I fasted from .... **until** ....

Total fasting period: ....

Today I moved by: ....
....
....

Today my blood glucose was: ....

REFLECTIONS

What I did well:
....
....

What I could improve:
....
....

Why today was great:
....
....

I'm not afraid of storms, for I'm learning how to sail my ship.
LOUISA MAY ALCOTT

DAY 5

How this quote applies to me: ....

....

Today I ate: ....

....

....

....

Today I fasted from .... **until** ....

Total fasting period: ....

Today I moved by: ....

....

....

Today my blood glucose was: ....

REFLECTIONS

What I did well:

....

....

What I could improve:

....

....

Why today was great:

....

....

You cannot change what
you are, only what you do.
PHILIP PULLMAN

How this quote applies to me: ....
....

Today I ate: ....
....
....
....

Today I fasted from .... **until** ....
Total fasting period: ....
Today I moved by: ....
....
....

Today my blood glucose was: ....

REFLECTIONS

What I did well:
....
....

What I could improve:
....
....

Why today was great:
....
....

Teachers can open the door,
but you must enter by yourself.
CHINESE PROVERB

How this quote applies to me: ....
....

Today I ate: ....
....
....
....

Today I fasted from .... **until** ....
Total fasting period: ....
Today I moved by: ....
....
....

Today my blood glucose was: ....

What I did well:
....
....

What I could improve:
....
....

Why today was great:
....
....

43

WEEK 3

Fasting: Increase your fasting window
and allow your body to use some of its
stored fuel (sugar and body fat).

My weekly goal—Fasting: ....

....

Today I ate: ....

....

....

....

Today I fasted from .... **until** ....

Total fasting period: ....

Today I moved by: ....

....

....

Today my blood glucose was: ....

REFLECTIONS

What I did well:

....

....

What I could improve:

....

....

Why today was great:

....

....

You never know when something
begins where it's going to take you.
JOAN W. BLOS

How this quote applies to me: ....
....

Today I ate: ....
....
....
....

Today I fasted from .... **until** ....

Total fasting period: ....

Today I moved by: ....
....
....

Today my blood glucose was: ....

REFLECTIONS

What I did well:
....
....

What I could improve:
....
....

Why today was great:
....
....

When you talk about something,
it's a dream; when you envision it, it's
possible; when you schedule it, it's real.

TONY ROBBINS

How this quote applies to me: ....

....

Today I ate: ....

....

....

....

Today I fasted from .... **until** ....

Total fasting period: ....

Today I moved by: ....

....

....

Today my blood glucose was: ....

REFLECTIONS

What I did well:

....

....

What I could improve:

....

....

Why today was great:

....

....

If it doesn't challenge you,
it won't change you.
FRED DEVITO

DAY 4

How this quote applies to me: ....

....

Today I ate: ....

....

....

....

Today I fasted from .... **until** ....

Total fasting period: ....

Today I moved by: ....

....

....

Today my blood glucose was: ....

REFLECTIONS

What I did well:

....

....

What I could improve:

....

....

Why today was great:

....

....

To change ourselves effectively, we first had to change our perceptions.

STEPHEN R. COVEY

DAY 5

How this quote applies to me: ....
....

Today I ate: ....
....
....
....

Today I fasted from .... **until** ....
Total fasting period: ....
Today I moved by: ....
....
....

Today my blood glucose was: ....

What I did well:
....
....

What I could improve:
....
....

Why today was great:
....
....

Success is the sum of small efforts
repeated day in and day out.
ROBERT COLLIER

How this quote applies to me: ....

....

Today I ate: ....

....

....

....

Today I fasted from .... **until** ....

Total fasting period: ....

Today I moved by: ....

....

....

Today my blood glucose was: ....

REFLECTIONS

What I did well:

....

....

What I could improve:

....

....

Why today was great:

....

....

Someone's opinion of you does
not have to become your reality.

LES BROWN

How this quote applies to me: ....
....

Today I ate: ....
....
....
....

Today I fasted from .... **until** ....

Total fasting period: ....

Today I moved by: ....
....
....

Today my blood glucose was: ....

What I did well:
....
....

What I could improve:
....
....

Why today was great:
....
....

WEEK 4

WEEKLY CHALLENGE
Movement: Move after every meal,
even if it is only five minutes of walking.
Allow your muscles to use some
of the glucose you just ate.

DAY 1

My weekly goal—Movement: ....

....

Today I ate: ....

....

....

....

Today I fasted from .... **until** ....

Total fasting period: ....

Today I moved by: ....

....

....

Today my blood glucose was: ....

REFLECTIONS

What I did well:

....

....

What I could improve:

....

....

Why today was great:

....

....

Do not wait.
The time will never be just right.
NAPOLEON HILL

How this quote applies to me: ....
....

Today I ate: ....
....
....
....

Today I fasted from .... **until** ....
Total fasting period: ....
Today I moved by: ....
....
....

Today my blood glucose was: ....

REFLECTIONS

What I did well:
....
....

What I could improve:
....
....

Why today was great:
....
....

A man can fail many times,
but he isn't a failure until he
begins to blame somebody else.
JOHN BURROUGHS

How this quote applies to me: ....

....

Today I ate: ....

....

....

....

Today I fasted from .... **until** ....

Total fasting period: ....

Today I moved by: ....

....

....

Today my blood glucose was: ....

REFLECTIONS

What I did well:

....

....

What I could improve:

....

....

Why today was great:

....

....

I just give myself permission to
suck... I find this hugely liberating.
JOHN GREEN

DAY 4

How this quote applies to me: ....
....

Today I ate: ....
....
....
....

Today I fasted from .... **until** ....
Total fasting period: ....
Today I moved by: ....
....
....

Today my blood glucose was: ....

REFLECTIONS

What I did well:
....
....

What I could improve:
....
....

Why today was great:
....
....

We cannot become what we need
to be by remaining what we are.
MAX DE PREE

How this quote applies to me: ....
....

Today I ate: ....
....
....
....

Today I fasted from .... **until** ....
Total fasting period: ....
Today I moved by: ....
....
....

Today my blood glucose was: ....

REFLECTIONS

What I did well:
....
....

What I could improve:
....
....

Why today was great:
....
....

Breathe. Exhale. Relax. Trust. Stop holding your breath, and allow life to take your breath away. You can surrender. You can let go.

MANDY HALE

How this quote applies to me: ....
....

Today I ate: ....
....
....
....

Today I fasted from .... **until** ....

Total fasting period: ....

Today I moved by: ....
....
....

Today my blood glucose was: ....

REFLECTIONS

What I did well:
....
....

What I could improve:
....
....

Why today was great:
....
....

Real change, enduring change, happens one step at a time.

RUTH BADER GINSBURG

How this quote applies to me: ....
....

Today I ate: ....
....
....
....

Today I fasted from .... **until** ....
Total fasting period: ....
Today I moved by: ....
....
....

Today my blood glucose was: ....

What I did well:
....
....

What I could improve:
....
....

Why today was great:
....
....

59

WEEK 5

Friends: Think of somebody
you are grateful for. Tell them
how much you appreciate them.
Phone, email, or send a message.

My weekly goal—Friends: ....

....

Today I ate: ....

....

....

....

Today I fasted from .... **until** ....

Total fasting period: ....

Today I moved by: ....

....

....

Today my blood glucose was: ....

REFLECTIONS

What I did well:

....

....

What I could improve:

....

....

Why today was great:

....

....

Today is hard, tomorrow will be worse, but the day after tomorrow will be sunshine.

JACK MA

How this quote applies to me: ....

....

Today I ate: ....

....

....

....

Today I fasted from .... **until** ....

Total fasting period: ....

Today I moved by: ....

....

....

Today my blood glucose was: ....

REFLECTIONS

What I did well:

....

....

What I could improve:

....

....

Why today was great:

....

....

People of accomplishment rarely sat
back and let things happen to them.
They went out and happened to things.
LEONARDO DA VINCI

DAY 3

How this quote applies to me: ....
....

Today I ate: ....
....
....
....

Today I fasted from .... **until** ....
Total fasting period: ....
Today I moved by: ....
....
....

Today my blood glucose was: ....

REFLECTIONS

What I did well:
....
....

What I could improve:
....
....

Why today was great:
....
....

You'll never find rainbows
if you're looking down.
CHARLIE CHAPLIN

DAY 4

How this quote applies to me: ....

....

Today I ate: ....

....

....

....

Today I fasted from .... **until** ....

Total fasting period: ....

Today I moved by: ....

....

....

Today my blood glucose was: ....

REFLECTIONS

What I did well:

....

....

What I could improve:

....

....

Why today was great:

....

....

Eat to live,
don't live to eat.

BENJAMIN FRANKLIN

How this quote applies to me: ....
....

Today I ate: ....
....
....
....

Today I fasted from .... **until** ....
Total fasting period: ....
Today I moved by: ....
....
....

Today my blood glucose was: ....

What I did well:
....
....

What I could improve:
....
....

Why today was great:
....
....

A goal is not always meant to
be reached; it often serves
simply as something to aim at.
BRUCE LEE

How this quote applies to me: ....
....

Today I ate: ....
....
....
....

Today I fasted from .... **until** ....
Total fasting period: ....
Today I moved by: ....
....
....

Today my blood glucose was: ....

REFLECTIONS

What I did well:
....
....

What I could improve:
....
....

Why today was great:
....
....

The time to relax is when
you don't have time for it.
SYDNEY J. HARRIS

How this quote applies to me: ....

....

Today I ate: ....

....

....

....

Today I fasted from .... **until** ....

Total fasting period: ....

Today I moved by: ....

....

....

Today my blood glucose was: ....

What I did well:

....

....

What I could improve:

....

....

Why today was great:

....

....

67

WEEK 6

Self-care: Take time this week
for yourself. Every day, take at least
fifteen minutes to relax and unwind.
Read a book. Go for a walk in the
forest. Take a bath. Meditate.

My weekly goal–Self-care: ....
....

Today I ate: ....
....
....
....

Today I fasted from .... **until** ....
Total fasting period: ....
Today I moved by: ....
....
....

Today my blood glucose was: ....

REFLECTIONS

What I did well:
....
....

What I could improve:
....
....

Why today was great:
....
....

No need to hurry. No need
to sparkle. No need to be
anybody but oneself.

VIRGINIA WOOLF

How this quote applies to me: ....
....

Today I ate: ....
....
....
....

Today I fasted from .... **until** ....

Total fasting period: ....

Today I moved by: ....
....
....

Today my blood glucose was: ....

REFLECTIONS

What I did well:
....
....

What I could improve:
....
....

Why today was great:
....
....

Yesterday is not ours to
recover, but tomorrow
is ours to win or to lose.
LYNDON B. JOHNSON

How this quote applies to me: ....

....

Today I ate: ....

....

....

....

Today I fasted from .... **until** ....

Total fasting period: ....

Today I moved by: ....

....

....

Today my blood glucose was: ....

What I did well:

....

....

What I could improve:

....

....

Why today was great:

....

....

Being defeated is often a temporary condition. Giving up is what makes it permanent.

MARILYN VOS SAVANT

How this quote applies to me: ....

....

Today I ate: ....

....

....

....

Today I fasted from .... **until** ....

Total fasting period: ....

Today I moved by: ....

....

....

Today my blood glucose was: ....

REFLECTIONS

What I did well:

....

....

What I could improve:

....

....

Why today was great:

....

....

A genuine fast cleanses
the body, mind and soul.
MAHATMA GANDHI

DAY 5

How this quote applies to me: ....
....

Today I ate: ....
....
....
....

Today I fasted from .... **until** ....
Total fasting period: ....
Today I moved by: ....
....
....

Today my blood glucose was: ....

REFLECTIONS

What I did well:
....
....

What I could improve:
....
....

Why today was great:
....
....

There must be quite a few
things a hot bath won't cure,
but I don't know many of them.
SYLVIA PLATH

How this quote applies to me: ....
....

Today I ate: ....
....
....
....

Today I fasted from .... **until** ....
Total fasting period: ....
Today I moved by: ....
....
....

Today my blood glucose was: ....

REFLECTIONS

What I did well:
....
....

What I could improve:
....
....

Why today was great:
....
....

Don't count the days;
make the days count.
MUHAMMAD ALI

How this quote applies to me: ....
....

Today I ate: ....
....
....
....

Today I fasted from .... **until** ....
Total fasting period: ....
Today I moved by: ....
....
....

Today my blood glucose was: ....

REFLECTIONS

What I did well:
....
....

What I could improve:
....
....

Why today was great:
....
....

WEEK 7

Sleep: Every day, make sure that you prioritize your sleep. It is a period of rest and recovery, and the lack of sleep has many harmful effects.

DAY 1

My weekly goal–Sleep: ....

....

Today I ate: ....

....

....

....

Today I fasted from .... **until** ....

Total fasting period: ....

Today I moved by: ....

....

....

Today my blood glucose was: ....

REFLECTIONS

What I did well:

....

....

What I could improve:

....

....

Why today was great:

....

....

Many of life's failures are people
who did not realize how close they
were to success when they gave up.
THOMAS EDISON

How this quote applies to me: ....

....

Today I ate: ....

....

....

....

Today I fasted from .... **until** ....

Total fasting period: ....

Today I moved by: ....

....

....

Today my blood glucose was: ....

REFLECTIONS

What I did well:

....

....

What I could improve:

....

....

Why today was great:

....

....

Fasting is the first
principle of medicine.
RUMI

How this quote applies to me: ....
....

Today I ate: ....
....
....
....

Today I fasted from .... **until** ....
Total fasting period: ....
Today I moved by: ....
....
....

Today my blood glucose was: ....

What I did well:
....
....

What I could improve:
....
....

Why today was great:
....
....

Marty, don't you ever
run away from a problem.
PHYLLIS REYNOLDS NAYLOR, *SHILOH*

DAY 4

How this quote applies to me: ....
....

Today I ate: ....
....
....
....

Today I fasted from .... **until** ....

Total fasting period: ....

Today I moved by: ....
....
....

Today my blood glucose was: ....

REFLECTIONS

What I did well:
....
....

What I could improve:
....
....

Why today was great:
....
....

A mistake is only an error.
It becomes a mistake when
you fail to correct it.
JOHN LENNON

How this quote applies to me: ....
....

Today I ate: ....
....
....
....

Today I fasted from .... **until** ....

Total fasting period: ....

Today I moved by: ....
....
....

Today my blood glucose was: ....

What I did well:
....
....

What I could improve:
....
....

Why today was great:
....
....

People are like bicycles.
They can keep their balance only
as long as they keep moving.
ALBERT EINSTEIN

How this quote applies to me: ....
....

Today I ate: ....
....
....
....

Today I fasted from .... **until** ....
Total fasting period: ....
Today I moved by: ....
....
....

Today my blood glucose was: ....

What I did well:
....
....

What I could improve:
....
....

Why today was great:
....
....

Fall seven times,
stand up eight.

JAPANESE PROVERB

How this quote applies to me: ....
....

Today I ate: ....
....
....
....

Today I fasted from .... **until** ....

Total fasting period: ....

Today I moved by: ....
....
....

Today my blood glucose was: ....

What I did well:
....
....

What I could improve:
....
....

Why today was great:
....
....

WEEK 8

WEEKLY CHALLENGE

Mindfulness: Practice mindful eating. Savor every bite of food. Don't eat if you are not hungry. That is your body telling you that it is perfectly happy using its stored energy.

DAY 1

My weekly goal–Mindfulness: ....
....

Today I ate: ....
....
....
....

Today I fasted from .... until ....
Total fasting period: ....
Today I moved by: ....
....
....

Today my blood glucose was: ....

REFLECTIONS

What I did well:
....
....

What I could improve:
....
....

Why today was great:
....
....

If you really want to do
something, you'll find a way.
If you don't, you'll find an excuse.
JIM ROHN

How this quote applies to me: ....

....

Today I ate: ....

....

....

....

Today I fasted from .... **until** ....

Total fasting period: ....

Today I moved by: ....

....

....

Today my blood glucose was: ....

What I did well:

....

....

What I could improve:

....

....

Why today was great:

....

....

What the eyes are for the outer
world, fasts are for the inner.
MAHATMA GANDHI

How this quote applies to me: ....
....

Today I ate: ....
....
....
....

Today I fasted from .... **until** ....
Total fasting period: ....
Today I moved by: ....
....
....

Today my blood glucose was: ....

REFLECTIONS

What I did well:
....
....

What I could improve:
....
....

Why today was great:
....
....

The credit belongs to the man who is actually in the arena... who strives valiantly; who errs, who comes short again and again, because there is no effort without error and shortcoming.

THEODORE ROOSEVELT

How this quote applies to me: ....
....

Today I ate: ....
....
....
....

Today I fasted from .... **until** ....

Total fasting period: ....

Today I moved by: ....
....
....

Today my blood glucose was: ....

REFLECTIONS

What I did well:
....
....

What I could improve:
....
....

Why today was great:
....
....

The greater danger for most of us lies not in setting our aim too high and falling short, but in setting our aim too low and achieving our mark.

MICHELANGELO

DAY 5

How this quote applies to me: ....
....

Today I ate: ....
....
....
....

Today I fasted from .... **until** ....
Total fasting period: ....
Today I moved by: ....
....
....

Today my blood glucose was: ....

REFLECTIONS

What I did well:
....
....

What I could improve:
....
....

Why today was great:
....
....

You don't drown by falling into water.
You only drown if you stay there.

CAVETT ROBERT

DAY 6

How this quote applies to me: ....
....

Today I ate: ....
....
....
....

Today I fasted from .... **until** ....
Total fasting period: ....
Today I moved by: ....
....
....

Today my blood glucose was: ....

REFLECTIONS

What I did well:
....
....

What I could improve:
....
....

Why today was great:
....
....

Weaknesses are just strengths in
the wrong environment.
MARIANNE CANTWELL

DAY 7

How this quote applies to me: ....
....

Today I ate: ....
....
....
....

Today I fasted from .... **until** ....
Total fasting period: ....
Today I moved by: ....
....
....

Today my blood glucose was: ....

REFLECTIONS

What I did well:
....
....

What I could improve:
....
....

Why today was great:
....
....

WEEK 9

WEEKLY CHALLENGE
Unplug: Take a break from social media this week. Instead, connect with your friends in person.

DAY 1

My weekly goal–Unplug: ....
....

Today I ate: ....
....
....
....

Today I fasted from .... **until** ....
Total fasting period: ....
Today I moved by: ....
....
....

Today my blood glucose was: ....

REFLECTIONS

What I did well:
....
....

What I could improve:
....
....

Why today was great:
....
....

Almost everything will work again if you unplug it for a few minutes, including you.
ANNE LAMOTT

How this quote applies to me: ....
....

Today I ate: ....
....
....
....

Today I fasted from .... **until** ....
Total fasting period: ....
Today I moved by: ....
....
....

Today my blood glucose was: ....

What I did well:
....
....

What I could improve:
....
....

Why today was great:
....
....

Everyone can perform magic,
everyone can reach his goal,
if he can think, wait and fast.

HERMANN HESSE

How this quote applies to me: ....

....

Today I ate: ....

....

....

....

Today I fasted from .... **until** ....

Total fasting period: ....

Today I moved by: ....

....

....

Today my blood glucose was: ....

What I did well:

....

....

What I could improve:

....

....

Why today was great:

....

....

If you want light to come
into your life, you need to
stand where it is shining.

GUY FINLEY

DAY 4

How this quote applies to me: ....

....

Today I ate: ....

....

....

....

Today I fasted from .... **until** ....

Total fasting period: ....

Today I moved by: ....

....

....

Today my blood glucose was: ....

REFLECTIONS

What I did well:

....

....

What I could improve:

....

....

Why today was great:

....

....

Impossible is a word to be found
only in the dictionary of fools.
NAPOLEON BONAPARTE

DAY 5

How this quote applies to me: ....
....

Today I ate: ....
....
....
....

Today I fasted from .... **until** ....
Total fasting period: ....
Today I moved by: ....
....
....

Today my blood glucose was: ....

REFLECTIONS

What I did well:
....
....

What I could improve:
....
....

Why today was great:
....
....

Success consists of going
from failure to failure
without loss of enthusiasm.
WINSTON CHURCHILL

How this quote applies to me: ....

....

Today I ate: ....

....

....

....

Today I fasted from .... **until** ....

Total fasting period: ....

Today I moved by: ....

....

....

Today my blood glucose was: ....

What I did well:

....

....

What I could improve:

....

....

Why today was great:

....

....

If you want to change attitudes,
start with a change in behavior.
WILLIAM GLASSER

How this quote applies to me: ....

....

Today I ate: ....

....

....

....

Today I fasted from .... **until** ....

Total fasting period: ....

Today I moved by: ....

....

....

Today my blood glucose was: ....

What I did well:

....

....

What I could improve:

....

....

Why today was great:

....

....

WEEK 10

Detox: Cut out all processed
foods for a week—no prepackaged
foods. Eat natural foods only.

DAY 1

My weekly goal–Detox: ....

....

Today I ate: ....

....

....

....

Today I fasted from .... **until** ....

Total fasting period: ....

Today I moved by: ....

....

....

Today my blood glucose was: ....

REFLECTIONS

What I did well:

....

....

What I could improve:

....

....

Why today was great:

....

....

You can't be that kid standing at the top of the waterslide, overthinking it. You have to go down the chute.

TINA FEY

How this quote applies to me: ....
....

Today I ate: ....
....
....
....

Today I fasted from .... **until** ....

Total fasting period: ....

Today I moved by: ....
....
....

Today my blood glucose was: ....

REFLECTIONS

What I did well:
....
....

What I could improve:
....
....

Why today was great:
....
....

Striving for success without
hard work is like trying to harvest
where you haven't planted.
DAVID BLY

DAY 3

How this quote applies to me: ....

....

Today I ate: ....

....

....

....

Today I fasted from .... **until** ....

Total fasting period: ....

Today I moved by: ....

....

....

Today my blood glucose was: ....

What I did well:

....

....

What I could improve:

....

....

Why today was great:

....

....

The only limit to our
realization of tomorrow
will be our doubts today.
FRANKLIN DELANO ROOSEVELT

DAY 4

How this quote applies to me: ....
....

Today I ate: ....
....
....
....

Today I fasted from .... **until** ....
Total fasting period: ....
Today I moved by: ....
....
....

Today my blood glucose was: ....

REFLECTIONS

What I did well:
....
....

What I could improve:
....
....

Why today was great:
....
....

Do you seriously believe anything worth-
while can be had merely for the wishing?
LLOYD ALEXANDER,
THE WIZARD IN THE TREE

How this quote applies to me: ....
....

Today I ate: ....
....
....
....

Today I fasted from .... **until** ....
Total fasting period: ....
Today I moved by: ....
....
....

Today my blood glucose was: ....

REFLECTIONS

What I did well:
....
....

What I could improve:
....
....

Why today was great:
....
....

The natural healing force
within each one of us is the
greatest force in getting well.
HIPPOCRATES

DAY 6

How this quote applies to me: ....

....

Today I ate: ....

....

....

....

Today I fasted from .... **until** ....

Total fasting period: ....

Today I moved by: ....

....

....

Today my blood glucose was: ....

REFLECTIONS

What I did well:

....

....

What I could improve:

....

....

Why today was great:

....

....

> Never allow a person to tell you no who doesn't have the power to say yes.
> **ELEANOR ROOSEVELT**

How this quote applies to me: ....

....

Today I ate: ....

....

....

....

Today I fasted from .... **until** ....

Total fasting period: ....

Today I moved by: ....

....

....

Today my blood glucose was: ....

What I did well:

....

....

What I could improve:

....

....

Why today was great:

....

....

WEEK 11

WEEKLY CHALLENGE
Small changes: Think about a tiny
habit you could implement to help
reduce the sugar in your diet.
Write it here:

....

Do it every day this week.

DAY 1

My weekly goal–Small changes: ....
....

Today I ate: ....
....
....
....

Today I fasted from .... **until** ....
Total fasting period: ....
Today I moved by: ....
....
....

Today my blood glucose was: ....

REFLECTIONS

What I did well:
....
....

What I could improve:
....
....

Why today was great:
....
....

The goal is not to be
better than the other man,
but your previous self.
THE DALAI LAMA

How this quote applies to me: ....
....

Today I ate: ....
....
....
....

Today I fasted from .... **until** ....
Total fasting period: ....
Today I moved by: ....
....
....

Today my blood glucose was: ....

REFLECTIONS

What I did well:
....
....

What I could improve:
....
....

Why today was great:
....
....

Fasting is a medicine.
SAINT JOHN CHRYSOSTOM

How this quote applies to me: ....
....

Today I ate: ....
....
....
....

Today I fasted from .... **until** ....
Total fasting period: ....
Today I moved by: ....
....
....

Today my blood glucose was: ....

REFLECTIONS

What I did well:
....
....

What I could improve:
....
....

Why today was great:
....
....

Change is hardest at the beginning.
But the good news is that it'll only
get easier. And you'll only feel better.
ROBIN SHARMA

How this quote applies to me: ....

....

Today I ate: ....

....

....

....

Today I fasted from .... **until** ....

Total fasting period: ....

Today I moved by: ....

....

....

Today my blood glucose was: ....

REFLECTIONS

What I did well:

....

....

What I could improve:

....

....

Why today was great:

....

....

If you are going through
hell, keep going.
WINSTON CHURCHILL

How this quote applies to me: ....
....

Today I ate: ....
....
....
....

Today I fasted from .... **until** ....
Total fasting period: ....
Today I moved by: ....
....
....

Today my blood glucose was: ....

What I did well:
....
....

What I could improve:
....
....

Why today was great:
....
....

I am a slow walker,
but I never walk back.
ABRAHAM LINCOLN

How this quote applies to me: ....
....

Today I ate: ....
....
....
....

Today I fasted from .... **until** ....
Total fasting period: ....
Today I moved by: ....
....
....

Today my blood glucose was: ....

What I did well:
....
....

What I could improve:
....
....

Why today was great:
....
....

Every strike brings me
closer to the next home run.
BABE RUTH

How this quote applies to me: ....

....

Today I ate: ....

....

....

....

Today I fasted from .... **until** ....

Total fasting period: ....

Today I moved by: ....

....

....

Today my blood glucose was: ....

REFLECTIONS

What I did well:

....

....

What I could improve:

....

....

Why today was great:

....

....

WEEK 12

WEEKLY CHALLENGE

Meditate: Sit quietly and comfortably
for five minutes each day. Close your
eyes and empty your mind. If stray
thoughts come in, gently push them
aside. Feel the calm, inner peace.

My weekly goal—Meditate: ....
....

Today I ate: ....
....
....
....

Today I fasted from .... **until** ....

Total fasting period: ....

Today I moved by: ....
....
....

Today my blood glucose was: ....

REFLECTIONS

What I did well:
....
....

What I could improve:
....
....

Why today was great:
....
....

Change the way you look at things,
and the things you look at change.
WAYNE W. DYER

How this quote applies to me: ....
....

Today I ate: ....
....
....
....

Today I fasted from .... **until** ....
Total fasting period: ....
Today I moved by: ....
....
....

Today my blood glucose was: ....

REFLECTIONS

What I did well:
....
....

What I could improve:
....
....

Why today was great:
....
....

I'm not in this world to live up to
your expectations and you're not
in this world to live up to mine.
BRUCE LEE

How this quote applies to me: ....

....

Today I ate: ....

....

....

....

Today I fasted from .... **until** ....

Total fasting period: ....

Today I moved by: ....

....

....

Today my blood glucose was: ....

What I did well:

....

....

What I could improve:

....

....

Why today was great:

....

....

Believe you can and
you're halfway there.
THEODORE ROOSEVELT

How this quote applies to me: ....
....

Today I ate: ....
....
....
....

Today I fasted from .... **until** ....
Total fasting period: ....
Today I moved by: ....
....
....

Today my blood glucose was: ....

REFLECTIONS

What I did well:
....
....

What I could improve:
....
....

Why today was great:
....
....

When someone tells me "no," it doesn't mean I can't do it, it simply means I can't do it with them.

KAREN E. QUINONES MILLER

DAY 5

How this quote applies to me: ....
....

Today I ate: ....
....
....
....

Today I fasted from .... **until** ....
Total fasting period: ....
Today I moved by: ....
....
....

Today my blood glucose was: ....

REFLECTIONS

What I did well:
....
....

What I could improve:
....
....

Why today was great:
....
....

Strength does not come from physical capacity. It comes from an indomitable will.

MAHATMA GANDHI

DAY 6

How this quote applies to me: ....

....

Today I ate: ....

....

....

....

Today I fasted from .... **until** ....

Total fasting period: ....

Today I moved by: ....

....

....

Today my blood glucose was: ....

REFLECTIONS

What I did well:

....

....

What I could improve:

....

....

Why today was great:

....

....

If you only do what you can do, you will never be more than you are now.
MASTER OOGWAY, *KUNG FU PANDA*

How this quote applies to me: ....

....

Today I ate: ....

....

....

....

Today I fasted from .... **until** ....

Total fasting period: ....

Today I moved by: ....

....

....

Today my blood glucose was: ....

What I did well:

....

....

What I could improve:

....

....

Why today was great:

....

....

APPENDIX: WHAT TO EAT

Adapted from Kelly Siverhus, *Low-Carbohydrate and Very Low-Carbohydrate Eating Patterns in Adults With Diabetes: A Guide for Health Care Providers* (American Diabetes Association, 2022).

ZERO-CARBOHYDRATE FOODS

MEAT
Beef

Lamb

Pork

Veal

POULTRY
Chicken

Cornish hen

Duck

Goose

Turkey

FISH/SHELLFISH
Clams

Crab

Lobster

Oyster

Salmon

Sardines

Scallops

Shrimp

Tuna

OTHER PROTEIN SOURCES
Eggs

Egg whites

VERY-LOW-CARBOHYDRATE FOODS

LEAFY GREEN VEGETABLES

Arugula

Chicory

Endive

Escarole

Kale

Lettuce

Radicchio

NON-STARCHY VEGETABLES

Artichokes and artichoke
  hearts

Asparagus

Baby corn

Bamboo shoots

Beets

Bok choy

Broccoli, broccolini, and
  Chinese broccoli

Cabbage

Carrots

Cauliflower

Celery

Chayote

Cucumber

Daikon

Eggplant and Chinese
  eggplant

Fennel

Gourd

Green beans

Green onions/chives

Greens: collard, mustard, and
  turnip

Hearts of palm

Jicama

Kimchi

Kohlrabi

Leek

Mushrooms

Nopales

Okra

Onions and shallots

Pea pods and pea shoots

Peppers: all kinds

OTHER FOODS

Almond milk

Avocado

Cheese

Olives

Tahini

Tofu

LOW-CARBOHYDRATE FOODS

NUTS AND SEEDS

Almonds

Brazil nuts

Cashews

Chia

Macadamias

Pecans

Pine nuts

Pistachios

Pumpkin seeds

Sesame seeds

Walnuts

LOW-STARCH ALTERNATIVES

BREADS

Cauliflower "pizza crust"

Cucumber

Lettuce wraps

Low-carbohydrate wraps

RICE

Cauliflower rice

PASTAS

Eggplant lasagna

Zoodles (zucchini or squash
  noodles)

Zucchini parmigiani

POTATO

Mashed cauliflower

CHIPS

Kale chips

Roasted seaweed

FLOURS (WHEAT-FREE)

Almond flour

Arrowroot flour

Chickpea flour

Coconut flour

COFFEE AND TEA

Coffee: caffeinated
and decaffeinated

Tea: black, green, herbal,
oolong

CONDIMENTS

Chili paste:
harissa and sambal oelek

Curry paste:
yellow, green, and red

Dijon mustard

Hot sauce

Miso paste

Tahini (sesame paste)

Tamari soy sauce

Vinegar: apple cider, red and
white wine, rice wine,
sherry

OILS

Coconut oil

Extra-virgin olive oil

Ghee (clarified butter)

Toasted sesame oil

Walnut oil

SPICES

Black pepper

Cayenne pepper

Chili flakes and chili powder

Chipotle powder

Cinnamon, whole

Cumin, ground and
whole seeds

Curry powder

Herbes de Provence
(dried basil, lavender,
rosemary, fennel, thyme,
tarragon)

Nutmeg, whole

Turmeric

LOW-CARBOHYDRATE
RECIPES

For these and many other delicious recipes, check out *The Diabetes Code Cookbook: Delicious, Healthy, Low-Carb Recipes to Manage Your Insulin and Prevent and Reverse Type 2 Diabetes* by Dr. Jason Fung and Alison Maclean (Greystone Books, 2021).

EGGS BAKED IN PROSCIUTTO CUPS

MAKES 6 SERVINGS

1 Tbsp olive oil

12 slices prosciutto

6 large eggs

Aleppo pepper or chili flakes (optional)

Salt and pepper

Chopped fresh herbs (optional)

1. Preheat oven to 375°F/190°C. Lightly grease a muffin tin with olive oil.

2. Line each muffin cup with 2 slices of prosciutto arranged in a crisscross pattern. You're trying to completely cover the inside of each cup so the egg doesn't stick to the pan.

3. Crack an egg into each prosciutto cup. Season with Aleppo pepper or chili flakes, if using, and salt and pepper.

4. Bake for 15–18 minutes or until egg whites are opaque and prosciutto edges have browned.

5. To serve, place on individual plates and scatter herbs on top, if using. Leftovers will keep well refrigerated in an airtight container for 5 days. Serve at room temperature or rewarm briefly in a microwave oven.

POACHED EGG ON CAULIFLOWER CRUST

MAKES 4 SERVINGS

2½ lb/1 kg cauliflower
½ lb/225 g Cheddar, Gruyère, or mozzarella cheese
5 large eggs, divided
Salt and pepper
4 slices prosciutto (optional)

1. Break cauliflower into florets and pulse in a food processor very briefly until it looks like rice grains. Don't make cauliflower paste! Grate cheese. Preheat oven to 400°F/200°C. Line a baking sheet with parchment paper.

2. Heat a large heavy skillet over high heat. Sauté cauliflower, stirring constantly, for 5–7 minutes. You're trying to dry-roast as much moisture as possible from the cauliflower. Allow to cool, then squeeze and drain cauliflower grains through cheesecloth or a clean tea towel.

3. Combine drained cauliflower with cheese, 1 egg, salt and pepper. Form mixture into four discs on the baking sheet. Bake for 17–20 minutes until edges are crisp and brown.

4. Bring two small pots or a medium saucepan of water to a boil. Turn down heat, make a whirlpool with a wooden spoon, and crack 4 eggs, one at a time, gently sliding each of them into the water (2 to each pot if using small pots). Set a timer for 5 minutes. When eggs are poached, carefully remove to a plate.

5. To serve, place each cauliflower crust on a plate and top with a slice of prosciutto, if using, and a poached egg. Season eggs with salt and pepper.

TOM KHA

1-inch/2.5-cm piece fresh ginger

2 stalks lemongrass

3 limes

1½ lbs/700 g boneless chicken thighs or extra-firm tofu

½ lb/225 g shiitake or oyster mushrooms

6 sprigs cilantro, for serving

6 cups/1.5 L chicken broth

2 cups/500 mL coconut milk

2 Tbsp fish sauce

Salt and pepper

Chili oil, for serving

1. Grate ginger. Bruise lemongrass with the blunt edge of a knife and cut into pieces. Zest 2 limes and juice one of them. Cut the unzested lime into wedges. Cut chicken or tofu into 1-inch/2.5-cm cubes. Roughly chop mushrooms. Pick leaves from cilantro stalks.

2. In a medium soup pot over medium-high heat, combine ginger, lemongrass, lime zest, lime juice, and chicken broth. Bring mixture to a boil, turn down heat, and simmer for 15 minutes. Strain through a fine-mesh sieve, discarding solids. Return broth to a soup pot.

3. Add chicken (or tofu) and return to a boil. Turn down heat immediately, add mushrooms, and simmer for 15–20 minutes or until chicken is cooked through. If you are using tofu, this step will take 10–15 minutes.

4. Stir in coconut milk and fish sauce just until heated through. To serve, ladle into bowls and garnish with chili oil and cilantro.

AVOCADO WITH TUNA SALAD

2 stalks celery

¼ red onion

6 sprigs flat-leaf parsley

2 cans (each 6 oz/170 g) tuna, packed in oil or water

⅓ cup/80 mL full-fat sour cream

2 large perfectly ripe avocados

Salt and pepper

Lemon wedges, for serving

1. Mince celery, onion, and parsley. You should have approximately 2 tablespoons of each, minced. If your tuna is water packed, drain it.

2. In a bowl large enough to easily combine the ingredients, flake tuna with a fork. Lightly fold in sour cream, celery, onion, and parsley. Don't be rough—you don't want to make tuna paste! Season with salt and pepper. You can refrigerate tuna salad, covered, for up to 24 hours before serving.

3. To serve, halve avocados and remove pits. Scoop tuna salad into avocado centers, spritz with lemon juice, and serve with a lemon wedge on the side.

OPEN SESAME BROCCOLI

MAKES 4 SERVINGS

1 large head broccoli
2-inch/5-cm piece fresh ginger
2 Tbsp toasted sesame oil
2 Tbsp tamari
4 Tbsp sesame seeds
Salt and pepper

1. Cut broccoli into florets with some stem still attached. Cut stalk into slender discs. Finely chop ginger. Preheat oven to 425°F/220°C. Line a baking sheet with parchment paper.

2. In a bowl, toss broccoli with sesame oil and tamari. Arrange broccoli in a single layer on baking sheet, season lightly with salt and pepper, and roast for 20 minutes. Turn broccoli florets and cook for a further 5–8 minutes or until deep brown in places and still tender-crisp.

3. While broccoli is roasting, heat a small nonstick pan over medium heat. Add sesame seeds and dry-roast for 2–3 minutes or until light brown. Be careful—sesame seeds burn easily.

4. To serve, spoon broccoli into a large serving dish and shower generously with toasted sesame seeds. Serve immediately.

SPEEDY SHEET PAN FISH SUPPER

1 red onion

1 lb/450 g slender green beans

4 Tbsp mayonnaise

4 tsp Dijon mustard

4 fillets (each 6 oz/170 g) haddock, cod, halibut, or swordfish

⅓ cup/30 g sliced almonds

1 lb/450 g cherry or grape tomatoes

2 Tbsp olive oil

Salt and pepper

1. Line a rimmed baking sheet with parchment paper. Cut onion into large chunks. Trim green beans. In a small bowl, combine mayonnaise and Dijon. Preheat oven to 500°F/260°C.

2. Place fish fillets on baking sheet with plenty of space between them. With paper towel, pat fish dry. Brush mayonnaise-mustard mixture over each fillet. Sprinkle with sliced almonds. Season with salt and pepper.

3. In a large bowl, toss green beans, onion, and tomatoes in olive oil to coat. Distribute vegetables around and between fish fillets. Season with salt and pepper. Roast for 10–12 minutes, checking fish after 8 minutes and moving vegetables around so they don't burn. Fish is ready when it flakes easily with a fork.

4. To serve, divide fish and vegetables among individual plates. Serve immediately.

CHICKEN THIGHS
WITH SPROUTS AND SQUASH

MAKES 4–6 SERVINGS

1 lb/450 g Brussels sprouts

1 lb/450 g butternut squash

1 onion

4 cloves garlic

1 lemon

4 Tbsp olive oil, divided

2 Tbsp apple cider vinegar

1 tsp cayenne pepper

2 tsp paprika

8 chicken thighs, skin on and bones in

Salt and pepper

1. Trim and halve Brussels sprouts. Peel and chop squash into chunks. Cut onion into wedges. Mince garlic. Slice lemon thinly. Preheat oven to 450°F/230°C. Using 1 tablespoon of the olive oil, brush a roasting pan large enough to hold (just about) everything in one layer.

2. In a large bowl, combine sprouts, squash, onion, garlic, and lemon slices with 1 tablespoon of olive oil. Season with salt and pepper. Transfer to roasting pan and roast veggies in oven for 10 minutes.

3. While vegetables are roasting, combine remaining olive oil with apple cider vinegar, cayenne, paprika, and salt and pepper. Coat chicken with olive oil–vinegar mixture. Turn down the oven to 400°F/200°C. Place chicken atop veggies and roast for a further 35–40 minutes until juices run clear when chicken is pierced close to the bone.

4. To serve, divide chicken and vegetables among individual plates and spoon pan juices over top.

BISON BURGERS

1 small onion

2 sprigs sage

2 Tbsp olive oil, divided, plus more to dress arugula

1¼ lb/565 g ground bison (buffalo), or ground beef

Salt and pepper

⅓ cup/80 mL mayonnaise, for serving (optional)

1 Tbsp hot sauce, for serving (optional)

4 handfuls peppery arugula (optional)

1. Dice onion. Pick sage leaves and slice; discard stalks.

2. Heat 1 tablespoon of olive oil in a heavy skillet over medium heat. Sauté onion for 10–12 minutes or until deep brown and starting to caramelize. Transfer onion to a plate and allow to cool completely.

3. In a large bowl, combine bison, onion, sage, and salt and pepper. Use your fingertips to gently combine burger ingredients. Don't compress or overwork the meat or burgers will be tough.

4. In the skillet used to sauté onions or a grill pan, heat 1 tablespoon of olive oil. Cook burgers for 7 minutes, then flip and cook for 5 minutes for medium-rare. Remove from heat, tent loosely with aluminum foil, and allow to rest for 5–10 minutes.

5. In a small bowl, stir together mayonnaise and hot sauce, if using.

6. To serve, mound some arugula, if using, on plates. Drizzle with olive oil and season with salt and pepper. Top with burgers. Dollop burgers with spicy mayo and serve.

MY
NOTES